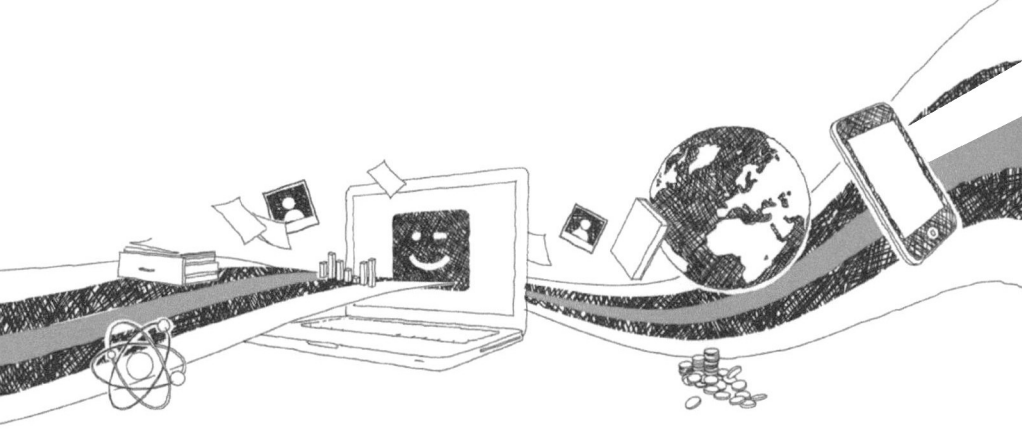
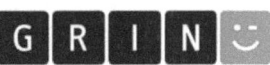

Mukasa Aziz Hawards

Fundamentals of the Human Body Immunity System

GRIN Verlag

Bibliografische Information der Deutschen Nationalbibliothek:

Die Deutsche Bibliothek verzeichnet diese Publikation in der Deutschen National-
bibliografie; detaillierte bibliografische Daten sind im Internet über http://dnb.d-
nb.de/ abrufbar.

Imprint:

Copyright © 2013 GRIN Verlag GmbH
Druck und Bindung: Books on Demand GmbH, Norderstedt Germany
ISBN: 978-3-656-53737-3

This book at GRIN:

http://www.grin.com/en/e-book/264197/fundamentals-of-the-human-body-immu-
nity-system

GRIN - Your knowledge has value

Der GRIN Verlag publiziert seit 1998 wissenschaftliche Arbeiten von Studenten, Hochschullehrern und anderen Akademikern als eBook und gedrucktes Buch. Die Verlagswebsite www.grin.com ist die ideale Plattform zur Veröffentlichung von Hausarbeiten, Abschlussarbeiten, wissenschaftlichen Aufsätzen, Dissertationen und Fachbüchern.

Visit us on the internet:

http://www.grin.com/

http://www.facebook.com/grincom

http://www.twitter.com/grin_com

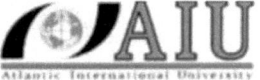

STUDENT NAME: **MUKASA AZIZ**

COURSE NAME: **Public Health Immunology**

Essay Title:

"**Fundamentals of the Human Body Immunity System**"

ATLANTIC INTERNATIONAL UNIVERSITY

October 2013

Atlantic International University
A New Age for Distance Learning

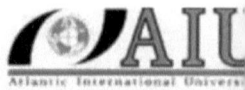

Table of Contents

Page

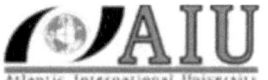
Course Description

Immunology as applied to public health. Emphasis is upon applications of immunology and immunological techniques used in surveillance, prevention, and control of public health problems.

The primary goals of this course are to familiarize the student with basic principles of, and recent developments in, the immunology of infectious and parasitic diseases and to develop a better understanding of the applications of immunology as a discipline in public health. Students who successfully complete this course will understand and be able to utilize the principles of detection, diagnosis, prevention and control of infectious disease through immunologic means.

Objectives

The learning outcomes of this course study include knowledge and understanding of a range of environmental topics as well as intellectual, practical and transferable skills and competences, as detailed below;

1. Understanding and apply principles of human immunology as it relates to infectious disease control in public health practice.
2. To proficiently apply fundamental principles of immunologic techniques to discriminate between and select appropriate methodology for diagnosis and prevention of infectious disease.
3. To comprehend with precise ability to compare and contrast the different immunologic reactions to pathogenic microorganisms in the human host and understand the relevance.

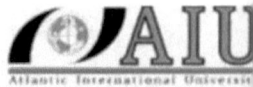

1. Introduction

In so many cases, we have been accustomed to the phrase "prevention is better than cure" yet in so many cases, we find ourselves as victims of disease that in so many instances, we are not sure how we came to contract them but instead the next step we embark on is to treat them.

It does not require extensive knowledge to realize that our body systems have inbuilt immune mechanisms by which humans survive the prevalent infections caused by the common bacteria located in almost every environment of man's involvement. The fact of immunity is not an artificial health aspect built on man's innovations in science but rather a natural fundamental of human life and therefore this provides the basis of preventive health and immunization.

Body immunity refers to the process or phenomenon through or by which the living body system is capable of identifying, isolating the foreign intruding harmful microorganisms and destroy or disarm them of the toxins that would be hazardous to the normal functioning of the body. The ability of the body to activate immunity against harmful microbes determines the health status of an individual and this is the foundation of immunology which is a perspective study directed against infectious disease spread in human communities.

Immunology, which is basic subject in medical sciences, finds its purpose along with microbiology, infectious disease control. In consortium with these medical subjects, immunology is regarded as the study of the fundamental physiological body components (molecules, tissues, cells, organs and systems) that are responsible of isolating foreign harmful bodies and disposing them out. The significance of immunology in the health science world is that it explores the common trends of disease emergence with an intention not of epidemiological importance but far more to devise vaccination, which can is applicable to prevent it from continuity.

The foundations of immunology can be traced from the early scientists such as Edward **Jenner** 1796, and **Neisser** 1879 that studied the response of the human body towards foreign organisms and the first inoculation of the human pathogen respectively. On to these contributors also pasture and the germ theory movement scientists can be considered as pillars in the establishing the basis and concepts of the subject of body immunity (York, 1996)

Through this conceptual and systematic study of immunology, the fundamental constituents of human immunity system, their functional pathways, regeneration, and replacement are analyzed. The study paper also entails the significance of immunology in the public health strategies of reducing health inequalities and disparities in the international community through international conventions on health policy structuring such as immunization are idealized.

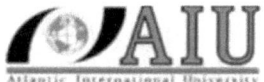
2.   Part I
Foundations and concepts of immunology

2.1 Historical Development

It was in the 19th centuries, the apocalypse period due to the deadly smallpox disease in Europe that Edward Jenner realized the ability of helping the body immunity system by artificial means to fight foreign bodies that could intrude into humans with infection i.e. bacteria. Jenner practically analyzed that the dairy maids had another form of cowpox which was of less danger at least with fatal end results as rapid as the smallpox and then by isolating this less weaker cowpox after obtaining samples from its victims.

Then the cowpox sample was latter introduced into the blood stream of normal individual from the hand and this caused blisters and scaly developments at the region of the skin from where the sample introduced. Surprisingly after two months the same individual was inoculated with the sample of the detrimental smallpox disease from patients and the results showed no devastating clinical effects in the tested person.

Onto this experiment it was idealized that the body had developed immunity to smallpox due to the fast infection of the cowpox which is almost of the same family. This also indicated that the body developed defending cells and anti-smallpox anti-biotics from within hence these were used to destroy the future patterns of the same likelihood.

The body was able to duplicate anti-bodies and anti-biotics of its own naturally using the post inflectional trends and hence therefore if all the disease pathogens can be inoculated in the laboratory by man then immunity will be a walkover. The disease causing pathogens are of different characteristics and these require different treatment for culturing artificially and this made more studies necessary in microbiology and serology. The experimental findings and achievements of Edward Jenner aroused more speculation and created more curiosity in the science field of disease treatment through which more discoveries were made by persons like **Neisser**.

By the year of 1879, Neisser was able to artificially isolate the first human pathogen gonococcus (EPHTI) and this achievement led to the production of the first definite human body antigen due to isolation of the diphtheria bacilli by **Klebs** and **Loeffler**. However, more scientific discoveries were made on disease and antitoxins that disarm the dangers of the pathogens in the body for the common disease trends of the time which also still today have a great significance in the medical field and health pursuits. The increasing discoveries by this time also called for more inventions of scientific tools such as microscopes and inoculating equipment in the laboratory field and more chiefly raised more awareness the cause of body immunity and how it works.

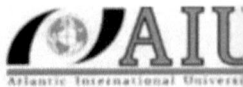
2.2 Rationale of immunology in health promotion

The epidemiology of the disease in the current world of health shows radical trends that must be interrupted or rather the hope of survival for the weak immune human systems should be forgotten. Nevertheless, this fact is proved by not only the explosion or emergence of new diseases but the fact that most of these disease pathogens are becoming more resilient even to the new drugs manufactured.

This is an area causing great threats and fear yet its effect is a silent killer that the world may take long to realize not until the scientific evidence for these possibilities and developments are made public for the entire world to know. The common diseases that used to be treated the normal traditional methods of common anti-biotics have strengthened and doubled in the resilience causing the need to develop better studies and discoveries through this kind of eruptions could possibly be terminated or averted.

More still, there is an increased emergence and eruption of mass killing or apocalypse epidemics most especially in the poor states and yet most of these are due to simple traits of pathogens caused by common problems of hygiene and nutrition. For instance, Ebola and cholera epidemics that erupted in the central and south central Uganda claimed the lives of innocent children and even health workers simply because the health sector was caught unaware hence the prevalence of the disease accumulated at unexpected degrees in the urban areas. What immunology does is to equip the health sector with the manual requirements and efficient technicalities in handling such scenarios after research thereby implementing preventive measures and immediate sensitization of the public. It is very shocking that the sensitization of the public about the sanitation causes of cholera was provided 3weeks after the eruption of the disease.

The World Health Organisation (WHO) and the United Nations Children's Fund (UNICEF) in the Alma-Ata Russia convention on world health programme laid strategies to combat health disparities in the international community and promote healthcare and nine strategies were identified to be chief capstones in this venture;

Objectives and strategies of the Alma-Ata Russia world health care convention (1978)

1. The availability and adequate access to water by the mass
2. Accessing safe sanitation
3. Adequate and healthy nutrition
4. Immunization against the killer diseases
5. Easy and quick treatment for cuts and common disease
6. Family planning advice, maternal and child care

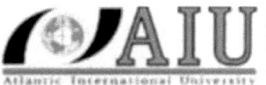
7. Public health sensitization or education in regard to healthy nutrition and preventive health methods
8. Advocacy for community participation in decision making in regard to preventive health planning
9. The training of village health workers to diagnose and proficiently treat common illness and injuries

This world healthcare convention aimed at achieving world health equality through the strategies by the year 2000 though one of the great blows that have tremendously compromised this plan is the eruption of new patterns and traits of disease infection.

Conceptually it can be postulated that health complications in humans are mainly of physical, infection and psychological which rarely claims life as compared to the former. However, among these, the infection factor contributes 89% of the hospitaliseable cables and yet some times the physical deformities lead to infection thereby indicating that almost 93% of the death cases are due to disease infection and the rest being accidental cases. This postulation is of great significance and it should be used to in order to locate and establish the role of the immunology paradigm in the pursuit of health promotion.

Most of the strategies that promulgated from the health convention places the prevention strategies to an Epi-center whereas those aimed at treating are regarded as secondary and policy oriented. On reckoning the national GDP for the majority of the states in the world it is discovered that 70 of these nations when picked at random at least lie below the poverty line and on estimating the economic statistics it is surprising to discover that 60% of the natives in such states have a very low gross per capita income. These individuals survive on almost 1$ per day or at least as less as 500$ per annum hence implying the treatment of even common diseases is not budgeted for yet when there is disease influx other utilities such as food, clothing have to be fore gone. This embarrassing economic status of the world's largest population is another cardinal factor that calls immunology preferably places immunology among the remedies that the world has to achieve health prevalence and enable sustainable development.

The naturally underlying foundations of body immunity such as breast feeding in the early infants and healthy diet or nutrition for both the adults and infants have been greatly decapitated from everyday life. The fact that the best a mother can give to the baby is breast feeding has become of no meaning and regarded as old fashioned method and replaced with food extracts from factories and others preserved with chemicals that will later achieve little in boosting efficient body immunity. This deteriorating trend can be attributed to poor and inadequate sensitization from the health sector about these fundamental health facts which has left the public ignorant and hence helping the prevalence of poor immune and disease infection.

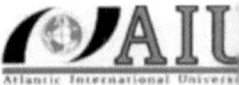
2.3   A Public Health Perspective in the Trends of Infectious Disease Prevalence

The notorious prevalence of infectious diseases have for the past centuries become an emblem of irresistible familiarity even to extent to extents total purging livelihoods in the prominent parts of the globe. Consider for instance the yield of the <u>Yersinia Pestis</u> that caused the extinction of almost a third of medieval Europe's total population from which the disease eruption was referred to as the "black death". Infectious disease also traversed across the military maneuvers in the ancient civilizations causing considerable due to diseases such as <u>Dysentery</u> and <u>Typhus</u> which once culminated into napoleon's retreat from conquering Russia after realizing that the effect of the typhus disease was even more devastating than the blows from the opponent forces.

In addition, the challenges can be remembered from the effects of the <u>Yellow Fever</u> which happened during the wars of French conquest in Cuba, the <u>Smallpox</u> invasions of the Europe's new world, <u>Malaria</u> infestation of the black continent that almost caused the racial and geographical patterns with the rest of the globe and so on. The list can stretch further even beyond unbelievable boundaries and the estimates of the number of death caused due to these disease emergences are in billions and billions across the offset generations of human existence.

Therefore, the shockingly high morbidity and mortality rates in the globe are caused by the infectious disease such as pneumonia which has been identified as the fifth leading cause of death among most disease yet and also leading among those connected to infection. It is estimated that by the year 2002, about 53 million deaths happened and estimated that at least 70% of these were due to infections.

These records are symbols of a worsening situation in the health aspects of our world and making it worse is the continual strengthening of the incurable diseases or perhaps those whose treatment vaccines have not been fully accomplished among which is the Acquired Immune Deficiency Syndrome (AIDS). The effects of the HIV/AIDS virus are of great far reaching extents and damaging not only the health trends all over the but also into other spheres of human involvement the worst has been felt via the social aspect. According to the word health report from the WHO in 20006 which was also the 25th anniversary for the AIDS epidemic it stated that almost 40million persons are living with HIV/AIDS and so far at least 25 have already died.

The African continent not only seem but it is actually the most haunted region of the international community by the HIV/AIDS stigma and the effects have been much felt in the sub-Saharan region and hence the leading cause of death. Other infectious diseases such as malaria are still in the region competing on scale against the AIDS stigma but while lagging due to the fact that their cure or treatment has been at least identified and this is not the fact with AIDS.

However, scientific companies and the pharmaceuticals have invented drugs that can control the virus trend but these drugs have nothing to do with the elimination of the disease though they can

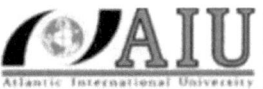
prolong the life span of the victims by temporarily boosting the body immune system. The ARVs are a mimicking of failure in curing the AIDS virus because what they achieve is to keep the body producing the anti-viral antibodies that sustain a periodical immunity that had previously been destructured by the virus.

Little has been revealed to the public about the AIDS virus but one of the key facts is that the virus is dynamic in structure. Therefore, while in the host the AIDS virus keeps on restructuring instantly hence making it hard for the body immunity system to duplicate the actual related and effective anti-body as it has always been with most of the previous infectious diseases.

The infectious disease can certainly be regarded as some of the common human health affiliates because the world we live in is a great sea of microorganisms even worsening still is that they still circulate in sterilized environments hence bacteria will take long to be eliminated.

3.   Part II
Principles in Basic Immunology and Inflammation

3.1 The Components of the Body Immune system
The common microorganisms that transmit or effect the prevalence of disease infection cannot be separated from the everyday environment hence the best way to achieve the prompt of minimizing disease spread is to devise scientific measures that are safe and applicable. The viruses, bacteria, fungi and parasites are the common wheels of infectious disease spread in the human physiology and leading to both less fatal and extremely fatal diseases contractions such as;

- Pneumonia
- Typhoid
- Streptococcal infection
- HIV/AIDS and tuberculosis

However, the natural immune system is designed structurally and physiologically to prevent the free intrusion and circulation of these pathogens in the living system and this is specifically carried out on two basic parameters i.e. destroying the foreign microorganisms and formation of the antibodies and the sensitized lymphocytes.

The mechanism of destroying the microorganisms is always the initial stage involving the detection of the foreign body or substance and after which immediate prevention mechanisms are undertaken by the leucocytes and the lymphocytes in eliminating, destroying or detoxifying it.

Formation of the immune anti-bodies serves to copy the structures of the pathogens by the body immune cells which after wards are capable of developing the resistant traits of blood

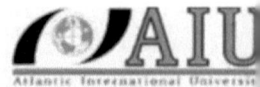
components that will effectively engulf and completely eliminate the pathogens. The immune system is mainly supported by the blood circulatory and lymphatic system that harbors the cell factors used in the role of fighting foreign microorganisms essentially recognised ones include the following outlined in the table below;

Figure 1: Table showing the major factors (types of Leucocytes) of the immune system in the blood and the lymph

Immunity Factor	Genesis Of The Factor	Basic Characteristics	Mechanism Of Activity
Leucocytes e.g. -Monocytes, -Lymphocytes -plasma cells - Polymorphonuclear Eosinophils - Polymorphonuclear basophils - Polymorphonuclear neutrophils	(a)Formed from the bone marrows (the granulocytes, monocytes, & some lymphocytes) (b) Moreover, others from the lymphatic tissues (plasma cells and the lymphocytic cells) (c) life span; -Monocytes: - 20hours in blood and 2months life span in tissues. -granulocytes:- 8hours in blood and 5days in the body tissues -lymphocytes:- weeks or months depending on body needs (d) monocytes and neutrophils are capable of squeezing into the blood capillary pores to join the body tissues (Diapedesis) (e) The Leucocytes move through body tissues by amoeboid motion. (alteration of body shape)	(a) Provide defense against infectious agents. (b) Detect and seek out the foreign intruder in the body (c) Some have granular appearance mainly the Polymorphonuclear traits. (d) A normal adult has about 7000 WBCs per blood microliter: Lymphocytes- 30.0%% Monocytes- 5.3% Polymorphonuclear neutrophils- 62.0% Polymorphonuclear eosinophiles- 2.3% Polymorphonuclear basophils- 0.4%	1. The granulocytes and the monocytes protect the body by ingestion of the pathogens i.e. Phagocytosis.

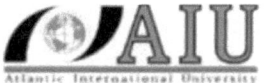
(f) Leucocytes locate the sources on detection of the composite chemicals and they are attracted henceforth by chemo-taxis.		

Adapted from: text book of physiology 11th edition by Guyton and Hall

The Neutrophils and the Macrophages

The macrophages are cellular derivatives originating from the monocytes, which turn on wandering in the body tissues after transition in the blood of about 10 to 20 hours. The monocytes while wandering in the body tissues swell into tissue macrophages and from this point, they start performing phagocytic mechanisms of eliminating the pathogens.

Both the neutrophils and the tissue macrophages are the major factors in the attack of the pathogens invading the body. The neutrophils are mature cells in the blood circulatory system and they directly attack and destroy the infectious bacteria in the blood stream whereas the tissue macrophages are immature cells and incapable of carrying effective immunity not until they reach the body tissues.

Cellular phagocytosis

This is the process involving the altering of the body shape and projecting the pseudopodia of the leucocyte, the intruding target microorganism is then engulfed and then destroyed from within.

Diagrammatic Illustration of Phagocytosis

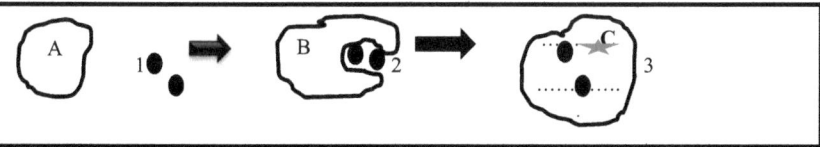

A. The leucocyte in proximity to the pathogens, **B.** the leucocytes alters the cell membrane and projects the pseudopodia to engulf the pathogen, **C.** The leucocyte completely invaginates its membrane to take in the pathogens into the endoplasm for ingestion
1. The foreign intruding pathogens in proximity to the leucocyte2. The pathogens are engulfed into the projections of the pseudopodia, **3.** The enveloped pathogens are digested by the leucocyte enzymes contained in the lysosomes of their protoplasm and the products released into the cytoplasm.

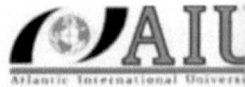
Phagocytosis is the major function of the neutrophils and the macrophages and they are suited for this function due to the following adaptations;

- They have extended and enlarged body sizes which they obtain after their transition from blood and as they join the body tissues. These sizes enable them to effectively and efficiently enclose the pathogens using the projections of their cell membrane.

- Their cell membrane is flexible and non-rigid as that of the cell walls in the plant kingdom. The flexibility of the membrane enables the leucocytes to easily alter their shape and form the projections that later enclose the pathogens during the process of phagocytosis.

- They have the lysosome enzymes in their protoplasm. The function of these proteolytic enzymes is to carry out the chemical digestion of the pathogens and detoxify their constituents. The macrophages mainly contain the proteolytic enzyme whereas the neutrophils contain vast quantities of the lipid digestive enzyme that breaks down the rigid lipid membrane of some bacteria.

- The leucocytes the neutrophils and the macrophages also contain the bactericidal components or factors which resume the combatting and killing of the bacteria if the lysosome enzymes are ineffective or absent. The main constituents of the bactericidal are oxidizing agents such as supper oxides (O_2^-), hydroxyl ions (^-OH), peroxides for example H_2O_2 and all these compounds are capable of digesting the tough protective coats of some bacteria that could not easily be digested by the lysosome enzymes. However, some special traits of bacteria are still a great challenge to this trend of digestion such as the tuberculosis bacillus that actually cannot be digested and these are causing synonymous eyebrows in the microbial laboratory fighting the prevalence of the infectious disease of tuberculosis.

The Eosinophils and the Basophils

The Eosinophils are very few in percentage as compared to other types of the leucocytes in the living body and though they are phagocytic in nature and mechanism their key role in body defense is minimal. They are of less effect in fighting body parasites due to their relatively small size in comparison to that of the majority of the human parasites hence they operate by attaching themselves to the pathogens and release substances which kill the disease causing germs. Clinical investigations shows that the Eosinophils are released in large quantities in the patients with parasitic infections for examples individuals with schistosomiasis commonly in the poor states of Asia and Africa.

Eosinophils attack the premature stages of the parasitic agents and they destroy them in the following mechanisms;

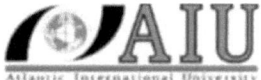
i.   Producing the extremely larvacidal polypeptide – major basic protein

ii.   Release of the hydrolytic enzymes from their modified lysosomes

iii.   Releasing of high oxygen reactants which are lethal to parasites

Beside the immunity role of the Eosinophils, they are capable of controlling the effect of inflammation though they perform this while in conjunction with the mast cells and the basophils.

The basophils on the hand are commonly circulated in the blood system and they locate themselves immediately at the capillary openings and they barely enter the body tissue. Along with the mast cells, the basophils are responsible for the prevention of blood coagulation and inflammation.

3.2 The Lymphoid System

The mammalian immune system mainly constitutes the lymphoid also made up of the special defensive cells called lymphocytes. It development is generated from the progenitor yolk sac cells and the liver in early stages of human development but later after a specified are is reached the bone marrows of the skeleton take on the production function for lymphocytes.

Primary and Secondary Lymphoid Organs

The lymphoid system is sub constituted of the primary and the secondary organ structures whose classification mainly depends on their role in the formation of the tissues that build the system and other accessory functions.

The primary lymphoid organs comprise of both the Thymus and the Bone which essential in providing the favourably tissue or microenvironments that promotes the emergence of the lymphocytes from the progenitor cells. Thymus is a gland located in the front of the heart and back of the sternum and its plays a role of proliferation and differentiation leading to the formation of the *Thymus-Derived T Cell*. However, the bone marrow is the main source of the progenitor or parent cells which later differentiate into lymphocytes, granulocytes, erythrocytes plus others and it also differentiates the B-Lymphocytes and cause bursa equivalence in humans.

The secondary lymphoid organs mainly acts as migration centers for the lymphocytes and functionally serves to maximize the degrees of encounters between the lymphocytes and the foreign substances in the body hence acts centers for launching immune responses. The main secondary lymphoid organs include:

Lymph nodes: - which filter the lymphatic system and instantly responds to the far antigens introduced or routed by afferent lymphatic.

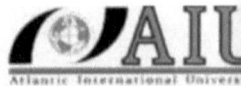
ii.   **Spleen**: - this accessory organ acts as the major site for antibody production that react against intravenous antigens e.g. bacteria. The spleen also acts as the lymphatic filter located within the blood vascular tree.

iii.   **The gut-associated lymphoid tissue**: - this organ consolidates the circulation of the lymphocytes particularly the B-lymphocytes from the payer's patches and the liver.

iv.   **Tonsils**: - these are located at certain levels of the lymphoid tissues as nodular aggregates and their principle role is to detect and respond to the invading pathogens in the respiratory secretion.

v.   **Blood**: - This is an important lymphoid organ that has an effective immunologic effect as a fluid tissue. The most important feature of blood is that it contains an efficient number of mature T-cells that release graft-versus-host reaction.

Lymphocytes

This is a special type of white blood cells that attacks the intruding of antigens according to a specific mechanism. The lymphocytes barely differ from each other may be by size and morphological features which can only analyzed under the microscope. They are grouped into three categories i.e. T-Lymphocytes, B-Lymphocytes and the Natural Killer (NK) Lymphocytes. The natural killer lymphocyte mechanisms and detailed features are quite extensive and due to nature of the topic it is not in the best interest to handle them briefly because that mighty mean less to science principles which have facts as the basis.

According to Goldman (Cecil medicine 23rd edition) it is postulated that all the lymphocytes both the T and the B are identical to each other in the amino acid sequence building. However, it is still stated that certainly not all the forms of lymphocytes are attracted to a particular antigen instead they have surface receptors, which are specific for the different antigens. Hence cloning for the lymphocytes depends on the progeny of the given cell, which express the same alongside the respective the receptor.

From the concept of the clonal selection theory, the cloning mechanism of the lymphocyte can be considered or better understood using an example of the mosaic shoe store with various sizes. Just as the design and size obtained depends on the specifications of the customer, also the cloned selection lymphocyte depends on the particular lymphocyte stimulated which later clones as controlled by the antigen (Immunology and Serology).

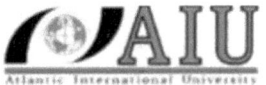
> ➢ **B-Lymphocytes**

These types of lymphocytes are the primary contributors towards hurmonal or antibody response that defend the body against harmful microorganisms. They originate from the parent cells via an antigen maturation independent process occurring in the bone marrow and the GALT.

Their operation is initiated after stimulation by the antigens towards which they respond by the secretion of Immunoglobulins and finally the production of antibodies.

Guyton, (2006) postulated that the hurmonal response of the B-Lymphocytes also requires the interaction between the macrophages and the T- cells and this serves to enable accurate detection of the antigen. According to Guyton, the role of the macrophages is to present the antigen cell to the T-cell and while using the surface bound receptor called the B-cell receptor, the B-cell recognizes its respective antigen after then it becomes activated.

Hence the activated B-Cell then possibly undergoes the process of cloning differentiates more into the plasma cells causing tremendous release or production of antibodies that fight disease infections in the body. However, the B-cells do not cross the line of plasma cells, at this stage they are always eliminated or excreted as worn-out antibodies, and they will barely be found within the blood circulation.

The B-Lymphocytes and the hurmonal immune response

The immune response mechanism is dependant on the nature of the foreign material in the successive stages of exposure. This can easily arouse or stimulate the B-cells even from their resting periods to enact them to enlarge, divide, mature and finally to produce antibodies.

The first stage of the immune response takes place at the debut of antigen encounter by an individual and at this point the immunoglobulin macrophage antibodies appear detectable in about 2weeks and after this, it declines leading to the secondary immune response.

The secondary immune response is carried out by the memory B-cells which becomes stimulated after the second antigen exposure of the same trait. The immunoglobulin-G is the major antibody produced during the secondary phase of immune response and it may prolong for long periods of time from months to years. This phase of immune response is attributed to be having extreme effectiveness and affinity due to the presence of the memory B-cells that actually are non-existent in the primary immune response phase.

Atlantic International University
A New Age for Distance Learning

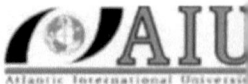

4.   **Part III**

Body Immunity: Types, and Factors for Effective Body Immunity

4.1 Types of Body Immunity

Scriver (2001) describes immunity as a process by which the body can protect itself when invaded or after the intrusion by disease causing microorganisms and at the same time devise defensive processes or mechanisms for preventing the harmful effects resulting from the activity of the pathogen. The immunity process involves both the prevention stage which comes immediately after the invasion of the antigens during which detection and identification of the antigen is carried out by the lymphocytes activated at the pathogenic arrival. However, if the immediate process stimulates effective immune response T-cells, then the pathogen action and effect are terminated immediately in which case few symptoms of the disease infection will be shown in the physical status of the individual.

However, in so many cases, this is not the case, rather the pathogen dominance might exceed beyond the initial stage of immediate termination but after being detected it prevails in the body tissue circulation. The cause of this possibility might be due to exposure nature of the immune system. For towards this particular or specific trait of the pathogen, for instance if it is the first time the body has been exposed to this type of pathogen then the cloning sequence and production of the necessary antibody may take long there by making the body system vulnerable to pathogenic prevalence. Secondly, if the "database" of the immune system has no previous traits resembling in structure the new intruding pathogen then the immunity may transcendently prevail to the secondary stage involving duplication of the likelihood of the antigen from the leukocytes.

Scientifically the immunity process has been categorised into two groups i.e.

❖ Nonspecific immunity
❖ Specific immunity

(a) Nonspecific immunity

This type of immunity can also be referred to as innate or natural immunity because it is inborn and not provided by artificial means. The natural immunity is the primary form of body immunity against disease infections and their respective pathogens and it serves to forfeit the intrusion and progress of the disease pathogens that have gained access to the body tissues. The natural immunity system ensures protection of the body against pathogenic effects by eliminating the microbes and neutralizing the toxic substances released by them through the following mechanisms;

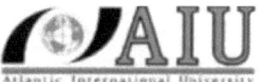
Physical or mechanical barrier formation: - The physical mechanisms of the body can be of great effect in ensuring the immunity pathogen invasions and effects. For example the skin, is a good barrier against microbe intrusion due to its moisturized nature, low PH and more so the presence of the secretory inhibitory substances (Baker FJ, 1995). Though it is very possible for microbes to intrude the body system through the hair follicles, sweat glands and sebaceous glands, this is however, partially prevented by the presence of further protective epithelia layers in regions such as the nasal cavity, respiratory and urinary tracts. Secretions from the barrier regions such as the mucus and urine are an added advantage for these parts to ensure effect removal of pathogens that had earlier penetrated into the body tissues.

Biochemical mechanism: - This preventive measure is founded on the body secretions that have negative impacts towards microbe colonies and succession in the host cells. The majority of the body fluids have inhibitory inductions on pathogens such as the hydrochloric acid in the stomach, bile juice in the duodenum. The tears from the eyes contain the lysosome enzyme that breaks down the cell wall of the gram positive bacteria due its hydrolyzing effect against the peptidoglycan layer (P.Stities Daniel. 1994)

Cell processes: - These processes are conducted principally by the neutrophils and the macrophages. The neutrophils ensures body defense by being the first factors to phagocytize the common pathogens at the infected body regions immediately whereas the natural killer lymphocytes conduct the killing of any undesirable cell e.g. tumor cells and the virus infected cells (Turgeon L.M, 1996)

The normal flora action: - The body flora consists of the non-harmful commensal bacteria colonies that occupy the attachment regions of the body tissues. These special traits of the of the body bacteria are important in the process of body defense by both competing for nutrients of nourishment with the pathogens and by releasing destructive substances against the germ cells intruding the body tissues.

The inflammatory mechanisms: - This is the immune response that involves the vascular and cellular reaction at the region of pathogen intrusion and possibly the most effective process in this criterion. Inflammation mechanism involves the stages of; (i). Tissue damage which initiates the immune response activity of the leukocyte against the intruding pathogen, (ii). Tissue response which is the activity of the stimulating the lymphocyte, (iii).leucocyte response which is a stage involving the confrontation of the lymphocyte supposedly phagocytosis in order to destroy and eliminate the invading microbe at the region. (iv). Tissue repair that constitutes the removal of the harmful and toxic substances from the region earlier infested with pathogens. (v). After the tissue repair stage then, the tissue regeneration or cure takes place. However, according

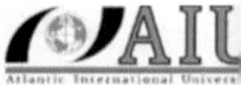
to Thomsen et al. (1998) the cure stage can be quite complicated due to the fact that not all cells types of the body are capable of regeneration. Take for example the skin cells which are comparatively suited for regeneration process and hence the cure stage won't be compromised as it have been the case if it was the nerve cells of the brain which are incapable of undergoing regeneration.

(b) Specific immunity

This is another type of body immunity system which is responsible for body defense against special diseases and common pathogenic infections. It can also be referred to as the adaptive immune response because it allows the body to adapt, remember and memorize and finally respond to a specific stimulating antigen. The foundational scholars in the paradigm of immunology discovered the ability of the body to identify the repetitive pathogens and while using this feature it was conceptualized that the body immune response system can certainly use this memory to produce antibodies. Further still, Goldsby (2003), describes the mechanism of the adaptive immunity system by asserting that it is operates on the immunologic memory and reinfection criteria in which case it could be the reason why humans might be victimized by some diseases such as measles once in the lifetime.

What adaptive immunity does is to immediately devise defensive mechanisms in the body, which alter the prevalence and progress of the pathogen either by phagocytosis or by release of destroying substances. However, in addition to pathogenic termination, the adaptive immune response system also keeps memory of that particular pathogen and builds up antibodies that will fight the antigens hence in future reinfection by the same microbe immediate termination of pathogenic dominance is carried out even before symptoms materialize.

However, adaptive immune response system can in one or the other be compromised for instance cases where individuals contract the same disease trait for more than one time as reportedly in the cases of malaria, fevers, influenza and cough. The reality of adaptive immunity cannot be disapproved at all costs even after such anomalies have characterized the health status of communities and therefore responsible for the shocking health disparities the fact remains that some diseases remain loyal to this rule of reinfection immunological memory response e.g. some of the immunisable killer diseases (Christensen et al. 1982).

Another form of immunity system has been conceptualized in the immunology paradigm as passive and this is obtained from the antibodies produced elsewhere after which they are fed into the blood stream of an individual. Passive immunity can still be further grouped under the following categories;

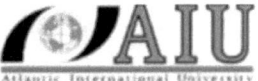
(i)   Natural acquired passive immunity;

This type of passive immunity is naturally generated from the mother and passed onto the fetus through the placenta as the channel. The placental region is highly vascularized with blood vessels and capillaries and these ensure the transfer of the blood and lymphoid constituents among which are the antibodies. Apart from the placenta the antibodies can also be passed onto the infants through the breastfeeding as newborns on colostrum and breast milk in the first 4-7 months of life.

(ii)   Artificially acquired passive immunity;

These are introduced antibodies formerly produced by an animal or a human. These antibodies are then introduced into an individual with an intention of pathogenic prevention and if not for purposes of infection treatment.

Active immunity: - This is contributed to by the physiological mechanism of the immune hurmonal leading to the production of antibodies in defense against foreign antigen. It can either be naturally acquired through the daily or common disease infections that cause the activation of the antibody production or artificially acquired due to vaccination.

4.2 Factors associated to immune response System efficiency

The individual immunity systems though they are morphologically and structurally identical due to the same genetic origin it has been investigated and experimentally proven that their efficiency from one person to another is considerably varying. The main reasons attributed to this phenomenon variation have been established on the facts of genetic difference and possibly which is responsible for the blood group patterns.

However, more evidence is evolving from health discoveries showing that some external factors that are particularly non-genetic have an impact on the efficiency of the immune system and these include;

(a) Age

The factor of age comparatively affects both the mature and infants concerning the immunity patterns. For example in the unborn and newly born infants the specific and the nonspecific immunity systems are possibly present they are still premature, less efficient and ineffective to prevent pathogens and destroy them from the body. not only the infants are vulnerable to disease infection and pathogenic attacks but also the old aged adults may face skin or physical barrier breakdown which on weakening opens accessible channels for pathogenic intrusion hence compromising the immunity efficiency(Turgeon L.M, 1996).

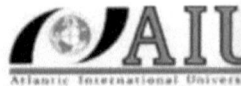
(b) Nutrition factor

Nutrition and feeding is a basic characteristic for all living organism because it supports the nourishment and proper progress for the rest of other body processes such as in respiration where it provides substances from which energy is released and in growth and development. Just like any other body system can be supported, the immunity system receives nourishment from the products of nutrition and hence poor nutrition implies inefficiency in the system and finally leading to poor health.

(c) Genetic disorders and determinations

Some diseases and health abnormalities are genetically controlled such as the sickle cell anemia, hemophilia, and so many others. In addition, due to genetic influence, the quantity of the body neutrophils produced can considerably be altered or even the multiple allele that are responsible for the blood group.

Scientific results from clinical investigations have shown that the individuals with blood group O are rarely affected by common diseases, as it is the case in those with A and B blood groupings.

4.3 Antigens, antibodies and the complementary system

4.3.1 Antigens
The antigens can be described as substances in the body whose presence and activity can stimulate the firing off an immune response action by the particular T-cell or any form immunoglobulin. In nature the antigens have got an epitope which is a site on their surface onto which the T-cell can attach itself and induce its immune response mechanisms. The antigens falls under the category of immunogens which are substances that generally triggers off the body immune response system and which include; bacterium, viruses and microbial pathogens.

However, Morowitz (1992), conceptualizes that not all antigens are immunogenic but their effect in body health can be determined on the factor of the number of epitope on their surface in which they are classified into multiple and monovalent epitope. Monovalent epitope is the situation where the antigen has only one site of attachment for the antibodies on its surface whereas multiples the sites of attachment are numerous. Therefore, depending on this characteristic it has been discovered and scientifically proven that antigenic molecules which have multiple epitopes induce strong immune body response than the monovalent traits.

In the medical field the antigens are used in the secondary prevention health approach where they help in the regeneration and rejuvenation of the immune system and along with this other substances called adjuvants are added to increase on the effect intensity of the immunogens. If the antigens cannot arouse the immune response system then the pathogens will easily enter and circulate throughout the body tissues without difficulty. Hence, while introducing an immunogen

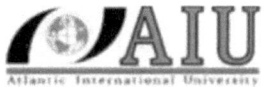
into the body it is important to combine it with an adjuvant, which accomplishes it, purpose as it cause the following;

i.   An adjuvant serves to prolong and lengthen the effects of the immunogen in the body

ii.   Maximizes the general increase in the size of the immunogens for effective identification by the macrophages and leukocytes

iii.   Increases the stimulation of the local influx of the macrophages and activates them for the preventive function.

Moreover, the immunogens qualify to their significance due to the contribution of the factors or conditions such as;

1. Chemical composition
2. Molecular size
3. Chemical complexity
4. Method of administration
5. Foreignness

4.3.2 Antibodies

These are types of glycoproteins that are secreted and sensitized by plasma cells and they respond towards special forms of antigenic stimulations in the body. Formerly the antibodies were referred to as gamma electrophoresis instead of the current immunoglobulin due to the first theory and observations that they were capable of mobility under gamma exposures but all this postulation the results have shown other traits of the antibodies which have no mobility under the gamma emissions.

The antibodies can be found in the different fluids of the body such as saliva, tears, and colostrum and in the plasma proteins of blood they form 20% of the constituent mainly in the serum or plod plasma.

Complete and incomplete antibodies

The complete type of antibodies can withstand high temperature fluctuations and on binding with the receptor sites or epitopes of the antigens, they can cause varying immunologic reactions whereas on the other side are the incomplete traits of antibodies.

The principle characteristic of incomplete or blocking antibodies is that they are easily altered by high temperatures and they are of less of completely no immunological effect or reaction when they bind with the antigen molecule. Unlike the complete traits of the antibodies which can penetrate through the placental barrier, the incomplete type of antibodies cannot by pass of penetrate the placental barrier. The different groups of antibodies have been outlined from

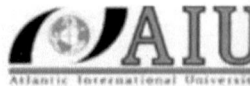
research due the mechanism of their operation when bound or joined with the antigens where as other aspects acting as basis for their classification include the following;

(a) Antitoxin antibodies which have and releases antitoxins to neutralize the poisons or toxins resulting from the antigens
(b) Agglutinin antibodies that immediately immobilize the mobile traits of bacteria and composes cell aggregates their by leading to the formation of clumps in which the bacteria are trapped and certainly rendered inefficiency
(c) Precipitin antibodies which react with antigen soluble molecules thereby forming precipitated complexes
(d) Opsonin antibodies that bind onto the bacterial surface and hence quickening the phagocytosis process
(e) Lysine antibodies which combine with the complement system to dissolve the antigen cell completely

4.3.3 The complementary system
This is a heat labile system of the nonspecific features which serve to amplify the specific functioning of the immune system and composed of about 18 series of plasma proteins. The proteins making up the complementary systems are always kept inactive however, during the a specific signal they easily get activated but in a systematic sequence.

The activation mechanism for this type of system is dependant on certain factors but the most postulated factor is the complex formation possibly of antigen-antibody molecule or in another way due to the presence of other foreign surfaces.

The activation of the complementary system

The activation process of this system follows two distinct routes i.e. the classic pathway and the alternate pathway. First of all the classical pathway follows a non-orderly sequence but from C_1 to C_9 i.e. $C_{1,4,2,3,5,6,7,8}$ & $_9$.

The complete alignment of the classical tree bases on the C_3 fixation which is actually existing within the plasma in very large quantities and since this pathway depends on the complex formation of the antigen and antibody molecule then it can be asserted that this is the principle feature setting up a line of difference from the alternative pathway.

The classical pathway is built up by three stages i.e. (i) recognition which is an enzyme interlocking level. (ii) the enzyme activation caused by the Clr and Cls (iii) membrane attack leading to cellular destruction cytolysis caused by the multiple actions of polymerization and membrane attack complex formation.

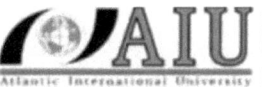

The alternative pathway however, is never initiated by anti-bodies which is one of its fundamental features separating it from the other pathway of complementary activation. This pathway indicates that only the microbial and the mammalian cells surface can possibly attribute to the activation of the complementary system and hence there will be no need for the antigen-antibody complexes.

Another fundamental property of the alternate pathway is that the tree or complete cascade of this pathway excludes the first three proteins (C_1, C_4 and C_2) and hence this implies that the protein C_3 will be activated by means of the complement proteins; factors B and D, which resembles C_2, C_1 and Properdin respectively.

Figure 4: The diagram below illustrates the complementary cascade: complementary activation pathways

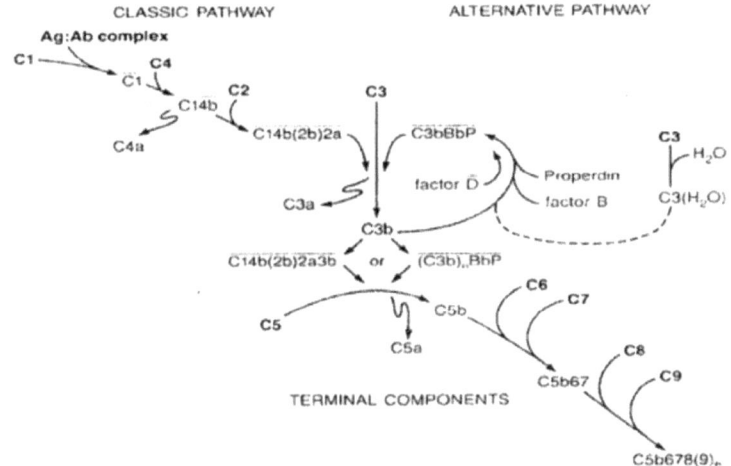

Source: Daniel P. Stites, et al. Basic and clinical Immunology, page 125

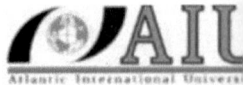
5.   **Part IV**

Key Aspects and Complimentary Aspects in Public Health Immunology

5.1 Preventive health care

Most of the strategies advocated for by the World Health Organisation (WHO) and the United Nations Children Fund (UNICEF) in the plan to promote health prevalence in the world's devastated regions such as the poor nations in Africa and Asia have concentrated on preventive measures and few have been directed towards treatment and cure of diseases. The prevention of diseases is of more value than the curing because the costs are reduced before the expenses are made on treatment of the diseases, which can even be resilient to the available drug, and hence more funds spent in research and development of more advanced drugs.

Preventive health care is a type of health care in the community either at work, school or at home, that is aimed at preventing disease prevalence rather than treatment or cure. The measures involved in preventive health care target the pre-infection and early infection stages of the disease in an individual and ensure that the victim or targeted person is exposed to the conditions that limit if not prevent pathogenic attacks.

The most haunting infectious diseases are possibly preventable actually the majority if not all the known diseases except the pandemic emergences such as the Ebola, cholera which in most cases catch the community unaware. But yet in consideration of the statistic for the mortality and morbidity rates of the world it shows that pandemics though they are spontaneous in nature, their claim over human death cannot be compared to the extent of the non-pandemic diseases. The largest numbers of death recorded are mainly contributed to by the infectious preventable disease traits such as the malaria common in sub-Saharan Africa, HIV/AIDS stigma still in Africa and other black communities both in America and in Europe, tuberculosis, pneumonia in the United States of America.

Further still preventive health care can be an advocacy campaign and policy aimed at raising awareness to the public about the possible outcomes of unhealthy activities such as smoking tobacco, excessive consumption of alcohol, having unprotected sexual intercourse, drug abuse and addiction, poor activity and inadequate nutritious diet. The preventive health care will design a random targeting pilot program aimed at sensitizing the community about the outcomes resulting from indulging in such unhealthy activities and by doing such, the threat of pathogenic infections might be reduced considerably.

Burtis (2006) describes the preventive health care paradigm as hierarchy process involving of systematic stages grouped into primary, secondary and tertiary preventive health care.

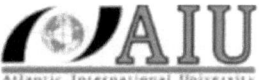
Primary preventive health care

This is the stage one in the preventive health care paradigm and it involves the implementation of disease preventive parameters in un-symptomized or individuals in whom expected disease signs have not yet materialized. The primary level of disease prevention outlines the unhealthy activities of the community and uses these orientations to predict the possible disease breakout in an individual or in the society.

In spite of the fact that the symptoms are not yet realized the role of the health technocrats and epidemiologist is to use the available channels of disease intrusion into the human community and this if carried out appropriately and under critical accuracy the possible disease infection can be averted and create a disease free community.

In the years between 2002 and 2010 the HIV/AIDS caused death have reduced tremendously in the Sub-Saharan Africa region by 60% as reported by the world Health organisation watch on the HIV/AIDS prevalence. In the early 2002 little sensitization initiatives existed and the civic education was only carried out the non-government organization while most of the regional governments paid a blind eye to such programs. However, the joint intervention of the World Health Organisation (WHO), USAID, and the involvement of the government agencies such as the health ministries added more fuel to the efforts of the non-government organisations by establishing more avenues of preventive advocacy for this disease in the community.

Strategies such as condom use for the unmarried couples, abstinence for the students, and faithfulness for the married ones have been advocated for. Through decampaigning against the sex networks in the community, individuals have resumed with living responsible behaviours make better relationship decisions thereby reducing their vulnerability to the contraction of the HIV/AIDS disease.

Secondary Preventive Health Care

This is a stage in the preventive health care process involving the immediate attending towards the early infection in an individual showing early and premature disease symptoms. During this stage, the early symptoms of the particular disease are identified in an individual which help the medical of the health workers to ascertain the type of disease and devise the early treatment or termination mechanism to prevent the progress and prevalence of the infection in the body.

Arend et al. (2007) describes the secondary stage as a screening level in a symptomized individual for the early detection of the preclinical disease risk before its propagation. It can involve the measurement of the serum lipid content in the droppings indicates the pathogenic intrusions and from this examination then effective antibiotics are applied to an individual for boosting and regeneration of the immune response system. In actual sense the secondary preventive health care stage has little if not nothing to do with the disease prevention because it

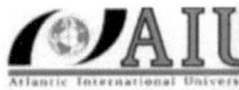
targets only the existing but un-established pathogen in the body tissues and if in any case it is not achieved the disease prevails hence causing devastating risks and dangers to the body.

The principle advantage of the secondary preventive health care stage is that the pathogenic colonies are still undeveloped and less effective hence can easily be disintegrated by the early application of the antibiotics used in the effective dosage.

Tertiary Preventive Health Care

This type of prevention is applied in the patient with known clinical complication with an aim of averting the effects and health risks of the disease. The disease infection has already undergone its successive propagative stages, circulated throughout the body tissues and blood stream, possibly weaknesses the immune response system and finally creates more pathogenic colonies without interference from the immune system. The table below shows a number of avertable death per year in the united states through the various prevention stages (figure2).

Figure 3: table showing the avertable death per year in the USA through the preventive health care

Preventive stage	Common infection	Avertable death per year
Primary preventive health care	- Pneumococcal vaccination of the elderly - Hypertension control - Reduction of total cholesterol by 10% - Physical activity - Smocking	- 9,922 - 68,382 - 132,777 - 177,940 - 328,044
Secondary preventive health care	- Pap smears - Fetal occult blood testing - Mammography	- 3,644 - 9,632 - 4,475
Tertiary preventive health care	- Warfarin after atrial fibrillation - Aspirin after acute myocardial infarction - β-blockers after acute myocardial infarction - Angiotensin-converting enzyme inhibitors for heart failure	- 3,418 - 10,365 - 17,023 - 11,000

Source: Woolf SH; The need for perspective in evidence-based medicine. JAMA 1999

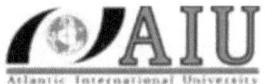
5.2 Strategic implementation of preventive health care

Preventive health care currently seems to be one of the principle tools through which health prevalence can be achieved in the international community due to the increasing uncertainty in the infectious trends and dynamics. The world is used to infections, they have stayed within the community of humans co-sharing the existence, and this discipline has enabled the development of the public health sector under stator and on the individual basis. Though infectious diseases have been co-existing alongside humans the fear is not their presence therefore, but instead their dynamic or changing traits which nowadays prove to be challenging in the pharmaceutical industry.

The malarial treatment drug commonly used in the world's stigmatized regions of this disease have always been undergoing periodical alterations not in dosage but shockingly in the chemical efficacy and constituent make up. New drugs on the drug shop have always been replaced and more over in a very short run of about 7-10 years by those seeming to be effective ones and more dynamic versions than the old ones.

However, this may sometime be mistaken to be resulting from new inventions and competitiveness within the pharmaceutical industry which at one point is true but not basically right. Why the human body would be turned into a marketing item or a fashion shop for drugs in just the prompt to get better sales and increase the company's interest rates as more public it attracted. But pharmacists are health workers who know the aggressive side effects resulting from the extensive consumption of even prescribed drugs in the human body and professionally they will always attend towards their code of conduct in which protecting human life at all costs is cardinal principle. The excessive drug intake is detrimental and has far reaching side effects which sometime may be fatal if not irreversible and this worsens when the body is exposed to new drugs without leaving an interval or refreshment and chemical elimination. These are possible problems known to the medical and health workers and for so many reasons such drugs have to be extensively studied and tested before being permitted to circulate to the public by the government.

The fact underlying the dynamic drug changes in the pharmaceutical industry for a single particular type of disease trait is that old drug versions have become of less effect. In other words the pathogenic traits have developed more protective mechanisms towards the drug, and in this case the pathogenic trait of that same disease therefore becomes resilient and this feature even increases with an increased dosage of the non-effective drug. The increased resilience of the pathogens towards the artificial immune applications such as vaccination and treatment have contributed to the need for developing the preventive health care units in the public health sector and this is more needful in the poor countries where the cost of living is very low but with high health costs.

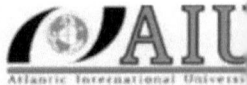
Further still, the hardest part in the paradigm of treatment and disease cure is the reality of high costs existing in the health and medical care both in the rich and the poor states. The costs of drugs are the same in both areas though the type of currency is the one altered from one part of the world to another. One of the many reasons that make the costs of medical and health care to be constant is that the poor states have not yet developed their home based pharmaceutical sectors and depending on the western world means, that all the prices will be controlled and determined by the same trustees.

Therefore, in order to escape the dilemma caused by the infectious treatment and disease cure there should be strong foundations created within the preventive health care unit through strategies and more importantly their implementation. The strategic implementation of the preventive health care unit can be obtained through some of the following channels;

1. Designing of prevention policies

The regional governments acting as the fore runners in the immunology paradigm should devise and structure targetful policies that can promote disease prevention in the community. The policies can in one way be statutory guidelines or legal landmarks enforced by the government agencies in private parastatals such as in schools, the media industry, health care centers and private hospitals, occupational health watch task force units etc.

For instance the government can "red-mark" some consumable products as health reduction and therefore such products if they are to be sold then the public should be warned about the possible dangers and resulting side effect from consuming them. These products may include both the addictive and non-addictive ones for example tobacco and coffee respectively.

Policies should be oriented in both ways of health promoting statutory guidelines towards the public communion sectors e.g. in schools and factories or they can be attractive (seductive) projects through media and other public centers.

2. Development of reminder systems in the health sector

Arend et al. (2007) states that "Patient reminders, either paper based (e.g., letters or postcards) or electronic (e.g., e-mail notices), can notify patients when preventive services are due and can help with follow-up on health behavior advice (e.g., reminding smokers about quit dates). Reminder systems are among the most effective steps that a practice can undertake to improve the quality of preventive care".

Preventive health care projects facilities such as the immunization season should be advocated for in the rural regions where health centers are rare and most of the babies are born outside the hospital. Such babies miss their health chances obtainable through immunization after birth and hence they are more vulnerable to infections of the seven killer diseases. However, through the

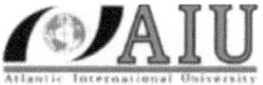
reminder systems, the possible effects of infection prevalence can be averted and the pulse for health prevalence elevated.

3. Practice redesign

The changing infectious disease trend is calling for a shift from the traditions to new preventive measures and strategies and thank God for the new technology and increased knowledge in science the world has a variety of choices through it pick the best method by which adjustments can be made to triumph over the increasing health disparities.

Preventive measures should be made easily accessible to the ordinary persons such that they can help themselves with the acquired knowledge about disease prevention even before the efforts of the medical and health service personnel are contacted.

5.3 The Public Health Capstone in the Immunology Paradigm:

5.3.1 Recommendations

According to Hamosh (2001), the breast-feeding process is the standard nutrition for the neonatal group of individuals because it contains many of the bioactive immune factors of the body that is still delicate. The concept is further supported by the fact that the neonates' immunity system is still incapable of withstanding the aggressive pathogenic colonies that may intrude into the body and hence an external supportive mechanism is required to rejuvenate and advance its efficiency. Unless breast-feeding is properly applied and adhered to by the nursing mother, the constant disease outbreaks in the lifetime of the child cannot be defeated completely.

Not only the idea of the neonates support the breast feeding as the principle foundation in body immunity but it is also true that the health person in adulthood depends a lot on the immunity foundation as laid by the breast feeding activity during childhood.

No wonder that even the frenzy pharmaceutical industries all over the world have developed their drug formulas with the highest components being derivatives of human breast milk in accompaniment with compounds such as polyunsaturated fatty acids and oligosaccharides but yet the public seem to have given this reality a blind eye. For the protein compounds contained in the breast milk as the principle constituent is also built from the combination of various bioactive factors such as;

- Immunoglobulins mainly the sIgA, IgG and less IgG that function by binding themselves onto the certain pathogens directly, adhesive binding and capable phagocytizing. Through these mechanisms, these bioactive factors modulate the local immune functionality and hence contribute to the proper functioning of the infant's immune system.

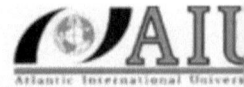
- Lactoferrin which operates by inhibiting the penetrative process of viruses, and contributes generally to the intestinal cellular repair if not growth.

- Lysozomes that causes the hydrolysis of the common bacterial cell wall their by weakening their protective coats and exposing them to easy attack by the antibodies

- Casein whose main role is to inhibit the occurrence of the adhesive characteristic for most of the bacteria in the epithelium of the various body regions and at the same time promotes the growth of the *Bifidobacterim*

The benefits derived from the breast-feeding process cannot be outnumbered by the contributions of the complementary drug prescriptions advocated in the globe today but due to lack of sensitization inefficient policy and strategy implementation, the public has diverted the natural attention towards industry products. No side effects throughout the generations have been idealized from human breast milk be it in concentration or in quantity. In other it is an immunity drug without prescription and yet not detrimental in whatsoever quantity it consumed in.

As discussed earlier that prevention not only saves life but it even spare the national economy by reducing the deficits in the national budget as caused by the treatment installations that are extremely expensive and financially unbearable to the poor communities.

There are so many factors and conditions that can be regulated at a cheaper cost by the government and yet their benefits are "unestimatable" in helping the promotion of preventive health care panoramas or projects. It is high time that the attention is focused on such factors such as public sensitization, occupational health inspection and establishment of disease screening centers with which the epidemiology of infectious disease is put to its maximum use in averting devastating health disparities.

Conclusion

The cardinal position of the immunology paradigm in public health promotion is the fact of health being a great resource and a basic row material in ensuring community development and fundamental change in the regions. For development to be achieved there must be a reliable assurance for an extended life expectancy in all the age groups both infants and the adults and this in the next point is only attainable only if the body immunity is effective and less vulnerable to infections.

The former scholars and scientists experimented with intention of discovering new trends of life to which human existence depended a knowledge which that was not in existence and end results

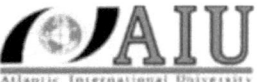

of the scientific explorations yielded the concepts that describe body immunity as a natural heritage for all individuals.

Perhaps with more efforts in the science of immunology there is another light at the end of the tunnel opening into everlasting hope of never to harbor incurable disease and that with such optimism the world labour tirelessly to curb the resilient infectious diseases such as the human immune virus disease (HIV) of AIDS. Not forgetting that programs developed under joint stakeholders have yielded more fruits that could not easily and quickly be attained under the individualistic aspects.

The main example can be borrowed from the reduced HIV/AIDS prevalence in the Sub-Saharan African region which has been a product of efforts from the world health organisation, the regional governments, humanitarian and other nongovernment sectors from the western world.

Bibliography

1. Arend armitage, clemmons drazen, griggs larusso; cecil medicine 23rd edition "an epert consult title: online + print. Published bysaunders elservier, j f kennedy boulvered 2007
2. Baker F.J. Introducion to Medical Laboratory Technology;6thed, 1995.Butter worth.
3. Blom, B., Res, P.C., & Spits, H. (1998) T cell precursors in man and mice. Crit. Rev. Immunol.
4. Brewster, J.H. (1986) Stereochemistry and the origins of life. J. Chem. Educ.
5. Bryskier A, ed. Antimicrobial Agents. Antibacterials and Antifungals, Washington, DC: ASM Press; 2005
6. Burtis CA, Ashwood ER, Bruns DE, ed. Tietz Textbook of Clinical Chemistry and Molecular Diagnosis, 4th ed. St. Louis: Elsevier Saunders; 2006
7. Christensen RD, MacFarlane JL, Taylor NL, Hill HR, Rothstein G. Blood and marrow neutrophils during experimental group B streptococcal infection: quantification of the stem cell, proliferative, storage and circulating pools. Pediatr Res 1982
8. de Jong MD, Simmons CP, Thanh TT, et al: Fatal outcome of human influenza A (H5N1) is associated with high viral load and hypercytokinemia. Nat Med 2006
9. Gesteland, R.F. & Atkins, J.F. (eds) (1993) The RNA World, Cold Spring Harbor Laboratory Press, Cold Spring Harbor, NY.
10. Goldsby, R.A., Kindt, T.J., Osborne, B.A., & Kuby, J. (2003) Immunology, 5th ed. W. H. Freeman and Company, New York.
11. Guyton. A.c and Hall. E. J: textbook of medical physiology 11th edition; published by elservier saunders jf kennedy boulverd, 2006
12. Hamosh M. Bioactive factors in human milk. Pediatr Clin North Am 2001.
13. Kotz, J.C. & Treichel, P., Jr. (1998) Chemistry and Chemical Reactivity, Saunders College Publishing, Fort Worth, TX.

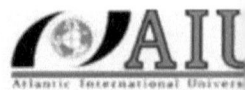
14. Morowitz, H.J. (1992) Beginnings of Cellular Life: Metabolism Recapitulates Biogenesis, Yale University Press, New Haven.

15. Scriver, C.R., Beaudet, A.L., Valle, D., Sly, W.S., Childs, B., Kinzler, L.W., & Vogelstein, B. (eds) (2001) The Metabolic and Molecular Bases of Inherited Disease, 8th edn, McGraw-Hill Professional, New York.

16. P.Stities Daniel. Basic and Clinical Immunology; 8thed, 1994,USA 4.Fischbach Frances, Manual of Laboratory and Diagnostic tests; 4ed 1992,Lippincott.

17. Thomas, P.J., Qu, B.-H., & Pederson, P.L. (1995) Defective protein folding as a basis of human disease. Trends Biochem. Sci.

18. Thomsen, A.R., Nansen, A., & Christensen, J.P. (1998) Virusinduced T cell activation and the inflammatory response. Curr. Top. Microbiol. Immunol

19. Turgeon L.M, Immunology and Serology in Laboratory Medicine,2nded, 1996,Mosby.

20. Van Parjis, L. & Abbas, A.K. (1998) Homeostasis and selftolerance in the immune system: turning lymphocytes off. Science

21. York, I.A. & Rock, K.L. (1996) Antigen processing and presentation by the class-I major histocompatibility complex. Annu. Rev. Immunol